SURVIVING CULTURAL STRESS

HELP! A ROBOT TOOK MY JOB

HOWARD MURAD, M.D.

Wisdom Waters Press
1000 Wilshire Blvd., #1500
Los Angeles, CA 90017-2457

Special discounts are available on quantity
purchases by corporations, associations, and others.
For details, contact the "Special Sales Department"
at the address above.

Printed in China

ISBN-10: 1-939642-22-1
ISBN-13: 978-1-939642-22-6

First Edition

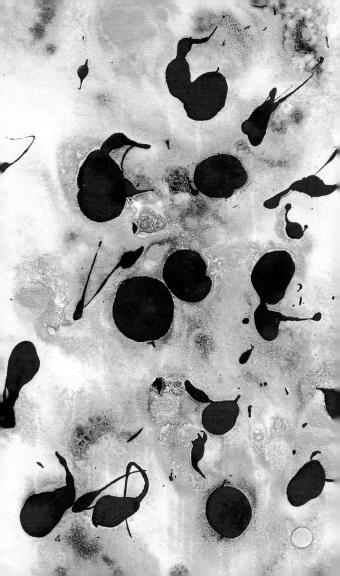

Life in the new millennium is generating a global earthquake of deadly stress and anxiety that is threatening each of us while spreading chaos throughout society. Here's how you can survive this crisis and enjoy greater health, happiness, and prosperity.

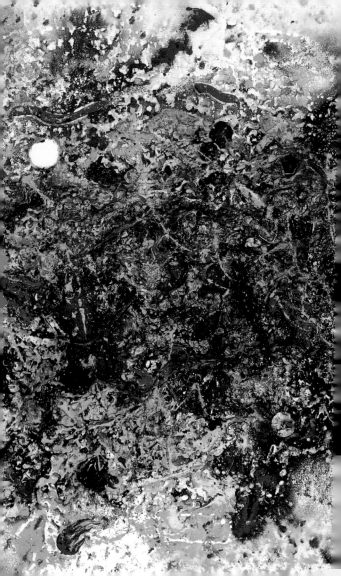

SURVIVING CULTURAL STRESS

People aren't talking *to* each other anymore. They are talking *at* each other. They are frustrated and dismayed, and their anger is spilling out into the streets. Some people say they can hardly recognize the world we're living in today.

What on earth is happening to us? The problem is at once quite simple and extremely complex. It's stress. But not that old-fashioned stress you feel when you're taking an exam, under pressure at work, or in the midst of an argument with a friend. No, this stress is a different thing altogether. It's *seismic*. Its sources run deep like the fault lines that produce major earthquakes. This new **Cultural Stress** is terribly dangerous and debilitating, and it's afflicting all of us.

Is Cultural Stress for real? Science says it is and it's deadly. More people die each year from stress-related illnesses than from any other cause. Most people don't even know they are suffering from Cultural Stress, making it a hidden affliction—a silent killer. It's stalking you, and if you have doubts about that, you'd better check your cell phone. You might have missed a text.

The communications explosion of recent decades has wrought social and political changes no less potent and stressful than those brought on by the industrial revolution two centuries ago. The jangling of cell phones is by no means the only way our 21st-century digital culture is poisoning us and our global society with stress. Today, information moves at the speed of light, and there's just no way to keep up with it. We want to answer every ring, text, and email and accomplish everything our culture demands of us. We strive for perfection, which, like a mirage, is always just out of reach. As a result, we feel at a loss, inadequate, overburdened, and cut off from our fellow human beings—even from nature itself.

In short, Cultural Stress is the constant, pervasive, and ever-increasing stress of modern living. It results not only from a dependency on digital forms of communication but from many other factors such as the growing financial pressures being placed on middle-class families, increasing expectations at work and at home, and a continuing surge in the rules and regulations we are expected to follow. It produces a condition I refer to as Cultural Stress anxiety disorder, which is associated with poor dietary habits, a sedentary lifestyle, loneliness, feelings of anger, and a diminished sense of self-worth.

What to do? Often, we can't change the factors that cause Cultural Stress, but we can change how we respond to them. We have to break out of our isolation, put away our perfectionism, win back the innocence and robust health of our youth, and start living again—*really* living. It's just as simple as that.

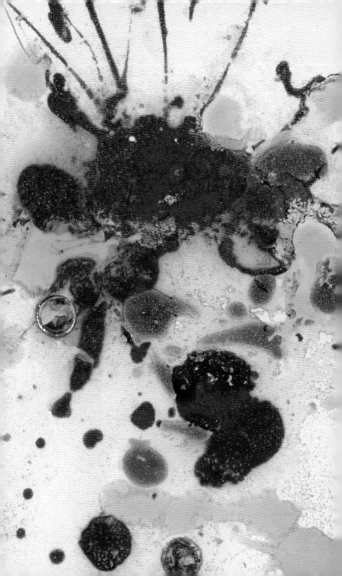

A ROBOT TOOK MY JOB

You know those times when you ask someone how they're doing and soon wish you hadn't?

My conversation with Jack was a little like that at first. He had made an appointment at my dermatology office in Manhattan Beach, California, so that I could treat him for a minor skin disorder. Thinking of it merely as a greeting, I asked the fateful question, and he immediately began to unload. For a while I feared he was going to relate his entire life history, and I really didn't have time for that. But the more I listened, the more interested I became in Jack as a person and in the story he had to tell. I found that it revealed a lot about the times in which we live—the troubled era of Cultural Stress.

"How am I doing?" Jack repeated the question. "I'll tell you how I'm doing. A robot just took my job."

"A robot?"

"You bet! I mean not one of those cute little guys you see in the movies, the kind with arms, legs, and eyes and who tell jokes but don't laugh. No, this robot is a lot more like an octopus than a friendly tinman, only this octopus has thousands of tentacles instead of eight, and they reach into everything, everywhere. The robot can do any of the things they used to pay me for and a lot more. I never had a chance. As soon as they had this thing up and running, they laid me off and several hundred of my friends."

Jack had worked in the shipping department of a large dotcom firm that sells books, computer equipment, clothing, food, wine, and "just about anything a person might ever want." Customers ordered online, choosing from among the countless offerings on the company's mammoth website, and employees like Jack packed their purchases in a box and shipped them. Or, at least, that's the way it had been done. Then the company found a way to automate the entire shipping process right down to the thank you card and the shipping label on the box.

"The funny thing about it is, the company computer guys used to come to me and ask me how we did this and how we did that," Jack said. "I explained it all to them, even the finer points that most people would never think about. For instance, you don't put plastic packing materials in with clothing orders. If you do, little bits of plastic will get all over the clothes and it's very hard to get them off even by washing."

"I didn't know that."

"Most people don't," Jack said. "But because I told the computer guys about it, now the robot does."

"You sound angry," I said.

"Yeah, I guess I am angry. I had a job and a life. Maybe it wasn't the greatest job in the world, but it was my job and I was good at it. Now I'm out of work."

Jack understood that the company was not entirely to blame for his predicament. After all, the company provided a decent severance package along with job counseling and a retraining program. Jack simply didn't find any of the training options particularly attractive. The company even offered to pay tuition for courses at a local community college.

"I'm just not the college type," Jack said.

Of course, it's impossible to see another person's life as they see it or to completely understand their motives. However, it did seem to me that Jack was closing doors before they'd had

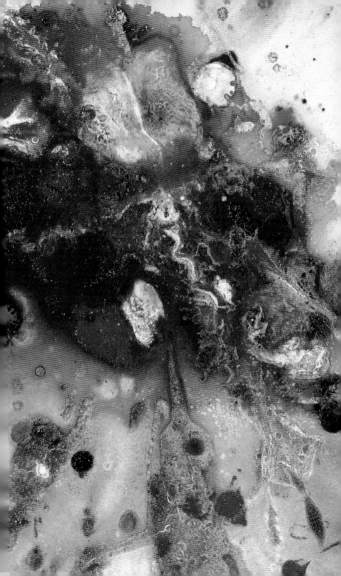

a chance to fully open. I wondered if Cultural Stress might be the reason.

"You've been under a lot of stress, I imagine."

"Stress?" Jack asked, as if the thought were totally new to him. "Yes, I guess so."

"After all, losing a job can be a terribly stressful experience, and anyway we're living in exceptionally stressful times."

Jack agreed that his life was stressful and had been especially so of late. We discussed how the stress might be affecting his skin condition, his overall health, his relationships with family and friends, and his day-to-day existence. Jack had plenty to say about all this. He was, after all, a very talkative fellow.

No matter how interested I was, I was mindful of other patients waiting and finally had to call our conversation to an end. We agreed that he would schedule a follow-up appointment for a few weeks down the line. As he left the office I gave him a copy of my book *Conquering Cultural Stress* (Wisdom Waters Press, 2015). He asked me to sign it and I did, adding the following as a postscript: *During your journey through life, expect to deal with change. Let it take you to new heights.*

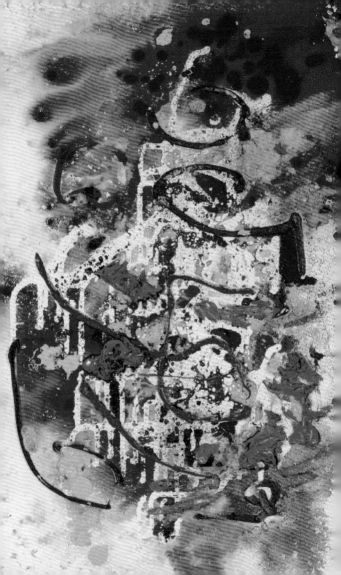

MARCH OF THE MACHINES

During the weeks after his office visit, I often thought of Jack and the predicament in which he had found himself. I marveled at his ability to bring a sense of humor to what for him was clearly an unfortunate situation. "The robot," that is what he had called the automated system that had replaced him and many of his fellow workers, and his description gave it life-like, almost human characteristics. Jack had smiled a bit when he made these comments, but I couldn't help wondering how much of this was a joke and how much of it truly represented current reality.

I decided to do some reading on trends in automation and the impact they are having on society. Some of my research was on the Internet—which has become rather robot-like itself, has it not? But I also paid a visit to an old friend: the UCLA library. All too often these days we tend to forget that real paper-and-print books can provide far more depth and context than any electronic database. Or maybe that's just my personal preference, but I've gone through much of my life with a book in my hand and some habits are hard to break.

What I have concluded is that robotic systems are no laughing matter. Robots are for real! And some of them are more than capable of tapping a worker on the shoulder and saying, in effect, "I'll take over from here."

The beginnings of automation can be traced back 200 years or more to the early days of the industrial revolution when machinery started

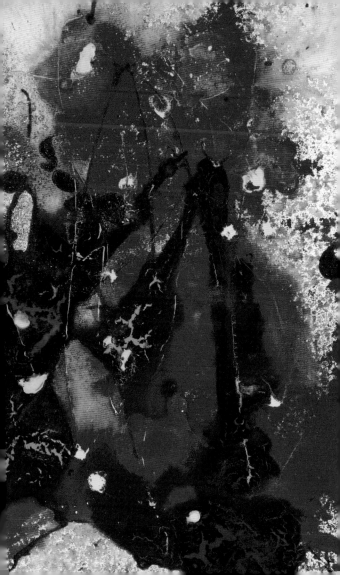

taking over repetitive tasks from human workers. Many people lost their means of livelihood and suffered great distress because of the mechanization of industry. But the new machines also increased productivity to such an extent that things got very much better. Living standards increased to levels that would have been unimaginable only a few decades earlier.

Perhaps the same thing is going on right now and we'll all end up very much better off and richer and as a result. Maybe, but the mindboggling sophistication of 21st-century machines place them in an entirely different category of invention than, say, a cotton gin or a steam engine. It's difficult to say for sure that the overall impact these machines have on people will be benign, and artificial intelligence adds a new and highly unpredictable factor. How long before we look at our ever-smarter machines and find they are staring back at us in soulless comprehension?

As daunting as all this sounds, there's really nothing much we can do to slow the process of automation, even if we wanted to do so. Automation is driven by economic and technological forces almost entirely beyond our control. Our machines and the computers that guide them will get "smarter," faster, and more capable no matter what we do, and if we get in the way and just stand there, they will run over us. What we *can* do is get out of the way! What we can control is how we as individuals respond to all these changes. And the best way to start is to reduce the heavy load of stress—Cultural Stress—generated by all these changes.

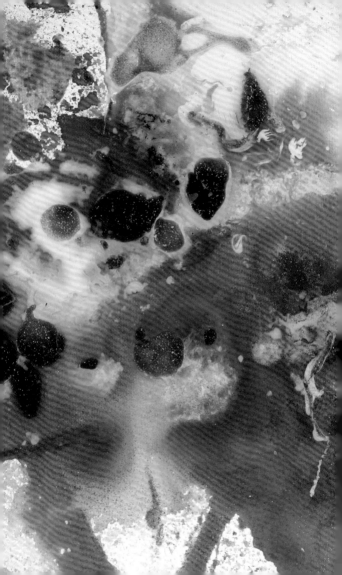

GETTING A HANDLE ON CULTURAL STRESS

learned a lot about Jack during his first visit. He was a strong-willed and creative man, and I was convinced that he would eventually find work. He was just not the type to let the machines keep him down, and he gave clear indications of this when he came to my office a few weeks later for a follow-up appointment. And not just because his skin condition had cleared up.

"There are a couple of things in here I wanted to ask you about," Jack said, holding the copy of *Conquering Cultural Stress* that I'd given him.

"Sure," I agreed, although I hoped we wouldn't be going through the entire book. That certainly seemed a possibility judging from the appearance of his copy which showed signs of heavy use. Many pages were dog-eared and passages were highlighted throughout with a yellow marker.

Conquering Cultural Stress is only a little more than 200 pages, but a book doesn't have to be a tome to have something significant to say. In the course of those pages I lay out my case against the silent killer Cultural Stress. It explains how Cultural Stress is generated by social media, cell phones, 24x7 news cycles, and the increasing isolation, financial pressure, and turmoil typical of modern life. I try to arm readers with ways they can defend themselves against the severe physical and emotional damage that Cultural Stress can cause. These defenses include an improved diet rich in structural water and embryonic foods, a more youthful and creative

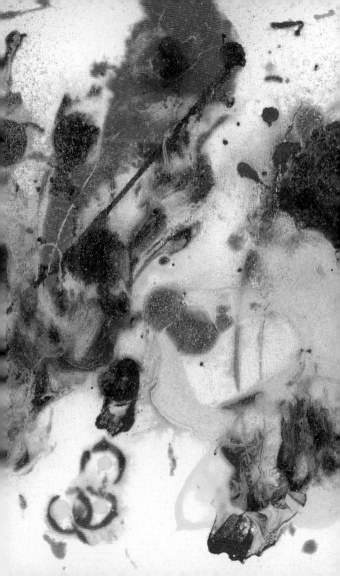

outlook on life, increased social interaction and exercise, and a willingness to abandon perfection as a goal. I thought these were the things Jack would want to ask me about, but he's a man full of surprises.

Jack turned to the back of the book and a list of brief insights I've had over the years. I included them in hopes that some readers may find them inspirational or possibly see them as a way to reduce stress. Jack pointed to this one: *Think of transition as an opportunity.*

"What did you mean by that?" he asked.

"Well, it means more or less what it says. Changes can be hard. They're nearly always stressful. But when things get shaken up, there are usually opportunities as well. Why not take advantage of them?"

"That's what I thought you meant," Jack said. "Thanks."

He shook my hand and turned to leave.

"Wait a minute," I said. "I thought you said you had a couple of questions."

"Nope, just that," he said as he went through the door.

THINKING ABOUT LIFE

It delighted me that Jack had found something useful among the insights listed in my book. The one he focused on—*Think of transition as an opportunity*—is among my personal favorites. But, over the years, I've composed hundreds of them. They're based on everyday observations I've made while treating patients, working with people around the office, or spending time with family. They're likely to pop into my mind at almost any time: in the morning while I'm having coffee, later in the day while I'm at work, when I'm having lunch or dinner, or just before I go to sleep at night. And if I'm able, when they occur to me, I write them down. They're just random thoughts I have that seem to me somehow likely to make it easier to live a healthier, happier, and more stress-free life.

By now I'd say I've collected at least 500 insights, and I keep adding to them. Why do I do this? Well, in part I do it for the same reason any writer writes—to express myself. But I also sincerely hope that someone like Jack will read them, take one or two of them to heart, and perhaps live a more fulfilling life as a result. However, you can never tell which of the insights will catch a person's eye or how they will respond to them. Here are a few of the insights that one might think would have appealed to someone in Jack's situation:

Life always throws curve balls; learn to hit them out of the park.

Allow hope to survive regardless of the circumstances.

Deal with what you have, not what you had.

It is not enough to know yourself, you need to become yourself.

Encourage your free spirit.

Give yourself permission to make your own journey.

Don't feel guilty for being yourself.

Don't just think out of the box; think as if there were no box.

Unlock your hidden potential.

Create new opportunities without fear of failure.

Real change only happens when you create your own.

Ultimately the impossible becomes possible.

The best is yet to come.

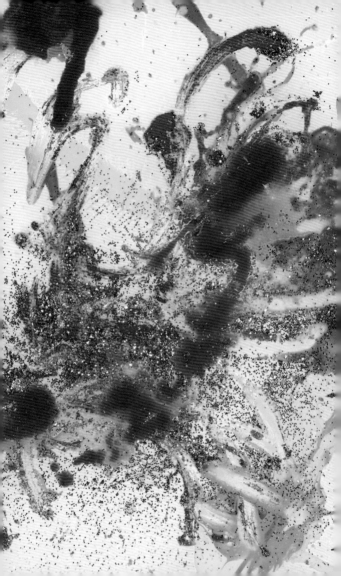

HITTING IT OUT OF THE PARK

I guess I'm not surprised that Jack took interest in an insight related to transitions. After all, he was faced with a big one and, no doubt, he was looking for options. I had no idea what he had in mind when he left my office after his follow-up appointment. I just hoped he had found my words encouraging.

Several months passed before Jack stopped by my office and asked if I had time for a quick chat. I made the time, anticipating that Jack would tell me he'd started a new career in a completely different line of work.

"Not long after my last appointment with you I went back to my former employers and told them I had an idea," Jack said. "Had they considered the possibility that some customers might prefer to have their goods packed by hand and that some might even be willing to pay a little more for the privilege?"

"What did they say?" I asked. This was intriguing and I could already sense where it might be heading.

"Frankly, I had expected them to laugh me out of the place, but they didn't. Maybe a couple of them smiled a little as I explained the concept, but they listened respectfully. Afterward we shook hands and they said they would get back to me. A few weeks ago, they did.

The company's marketing department tested Jack's idea and discovered that, indeed, many of their customers liked the idea of having their purchases pack by human hands rather than by a machine. They decided to offer hand packing

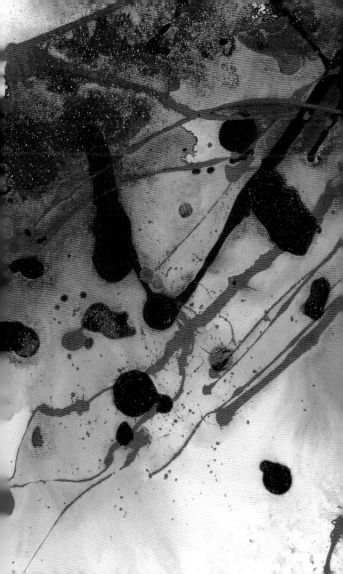

as an option but not to charge for it. Once they'd made a purchase, customers could click on a button that said "pack by hand."

So what did Jack get out of this? Well, for one thing a very welcome check and for another a new job. But instead of actually picking and packing orders as he had for so many years, he was hired on as a special customer service expert to help the company develop new and innovative offerings.

"Jack, that's terrific!" I said. "That's really thinking out of the box."

"No," he said, "that's thinking as if there were no box."

ABOUT THE ART

When I create paintings like the ones you see in this book, I make a few marks on canvas, add some colors, and spray them with water. The water interacts with the colors in a more or less random way, and this often carries the artwork in a totally unexpected direction. How's it going to turn out? I don't know.

My life has been like that too. Some might be surprised to learn that I started out thinking I wanted to be an engineer. When that didn't work out for me, I went into pharmacy and that, in turn, led me into medicine. Whatever happened along the way, I always felt life was carrying me somewhere. Life is a canvas, you see. You make your mark on it and then flow with it.

If you allow it to flow in a way that makes sense, your life will be a work of art.

Interestingly, I didn't start painting until 2008 when retinal surgery forced me to spend a rather challenging month always looking down. My wife, Loralee, suggested I try my hand at art to help me pass the time. I followed her advice and found that expressing myself with color on canvas was far more invigorating than I had ever imagined. I truly believe the painting helped me heal faster, and after that experience, I began to incorporate art into my overall skincare and general health philosophies. Along with an emphasis on personal creativity, my approach includes a diet rich in water and whole foods, appropriate skincare products, targeted supplements, rest, and plenty of exercise.

It also includes a positive attitude. If you smile a lot, you're going to look a lot more attractive. There is an emotional component to both your

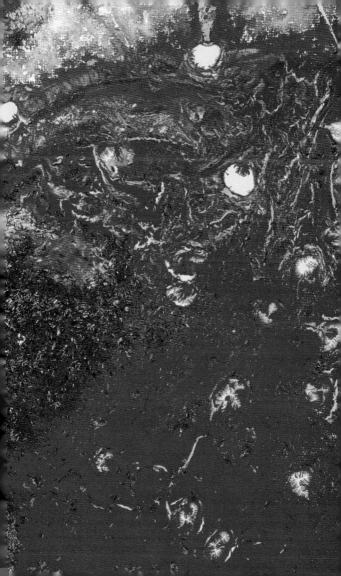

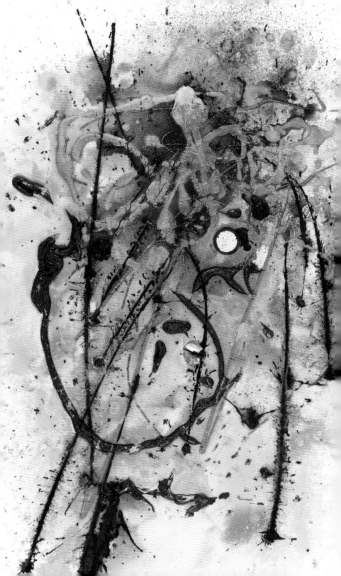

appearance and your health, and when you are creative your emotions are allowed to run free. If you have an engaging outlet for your natural creativity, you will sleep better, be more vibrant, and experience more happiness.

When I consult with patients, we don't just talk about individual skin conditions. These are always linked to other problems and concerns, so we discuss a whole range of health-related issues. We also discuss various ways people can express themselves creatively. What this comes down to in the end is finding ways to access their inner toddler, to look at the world around them the same way they did when they were just two or three years old. The freedom that comes with rediscovering that fresh, child-like outlook has benefits that extend far beyond art. It can improve every aspect of our existence, changing life into the youthful adventure it was always meant to be. That is why I always try to send my patients home with a plan that takes personal creativity into consideration. Art therapy works, and more and more hospitals and clinics are using it to improve both the emotional and physical health of their patients. I do the same in my medical practice and my writing. I especially encourage you to let the light of youth enter and make your own life a work of art.

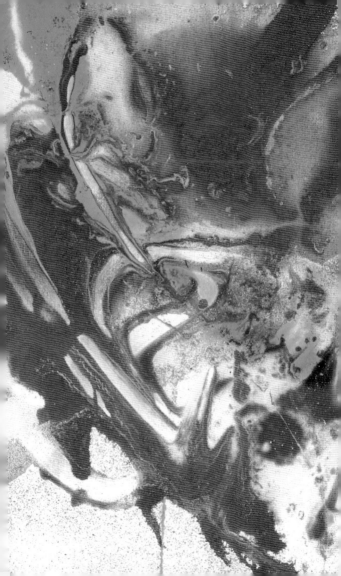

DR. HOWARD MURAD'S CONNECTED BEAUTY APPROACH

A prominent Los Angeles physician, Dr. Howard Murad has successfully treated more than 50,000 patients. Drawing on his training in both pharmacy and medicine, he has developed a popular and highly effective line of skincare products that has won praise from health and beauty conscious people everywhere. A practitioner not just of medicine but of the philosophy of health, he has written dozens of books and articles, and these have earned him a worldwide reputation as an authority on slowing the aging process.

Dr. Murad's approach to medicine is unique. It involves a concept he calls **Connected Beauty**. In the past he has referred to this same ground-breaking concept as Connected Health or Inclusive Health, but all these terms basically mean the same thing: Our skin, internal organs, diet, lifestyle, and fundamental outlook are very closely linked.

An alternative to traditional medical practice with its emphasis on the spot treatment of individual conditions or illnesses, the Connected Beauty philosophy is centered on the idea that healthy, beautiful skin is a reflection of how you live your life. Every aspect of your life directly affects cellular hydration and the health of every cell in your body. That is why Dr. Murad believes there is a powerful yet often overlooked connection between the mind, body, and skin. This link is the essence of the Connected Beauty concept which he has made the foundation of his whole-person approach to beauty, health,

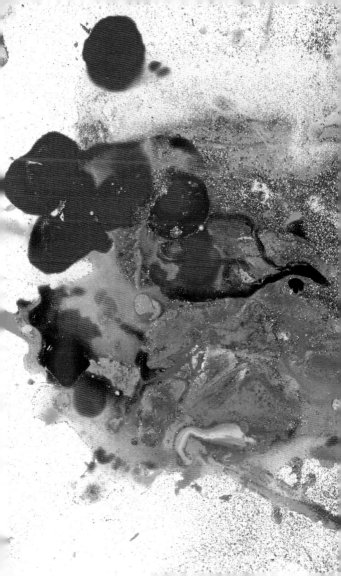

and well-being. It is intended to inspire you to take care of your skin not only with his highly effective products but also with proper nutrition, physical activity, and stress management.

Years of painstaking research and experience with thousands of patients have shown Dr. Murad that human health and happiness are, in fact, directly linked to the ability of cells to retain water. A poor diet and the stress of day-to-day living can damage the all-important membranes that form cell walls. Over time, these membranes become broken and porous, causing the cells to leak water and lose vitality. This, in turn, leads to accelerated aging and a wide variety of diseases and syndromes.

In his bestseller *The Water Secret*, published in 2010, Dr. Murad explained how to stop this process—and reverse it—through Inclusive or Connected Healthcare. This approach has three essential components. The first is a healthy diet that emphasizes raw fruits and vegetables. This allows us to literally eat the water our cells need to survive. Proper hydration levels cannot be maintained merely by drinking liquids, which pass right through our body while providing very little benefit. Instead, we must hydrate our cells by eating water-rich foods. The second component involves good skincare practices, and the third an overall reduction in stress combined with a more youthful and creative outlook on life.

The third component, which emphasizes our emotional state, may be the hardest part of the Connected Beauty treatment process for people to adopt. The breakneck pace of modern life with its freeways, computers, cell phones, and fast-paced living places upon us an enormous amount of what Dr. Murad describes as Cultural Stress. To deal with this runaway stress, we live increasingly structured lives that are less and less open to the free play and creativity that make life worth living.

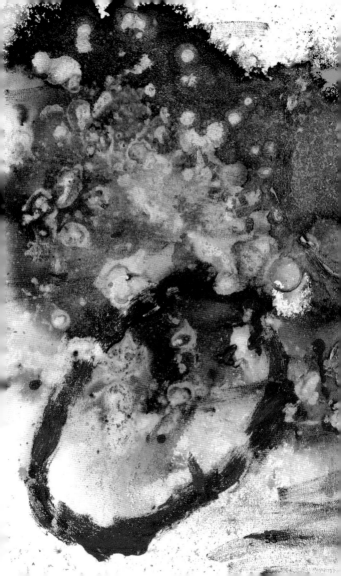

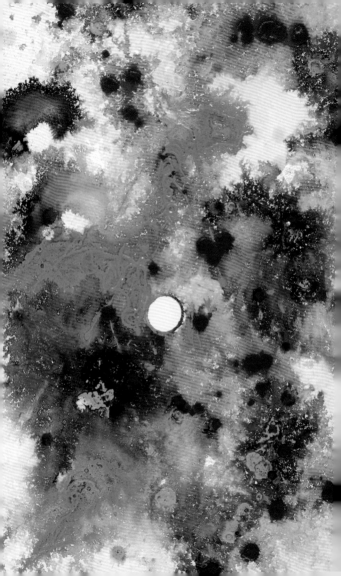

We can choose not to live this way. But reducing stress and embracing a more youthful outlook often involves major shifts in lifestyle: changes in jobs, accommodations, locales, hobbies, habits, and relationships. It may even require a complete personal transformation of the sort sometimes identified with a single galvanizing moment of self-awareness. You may experience a transforming moment like that while walking on a beach, creating a work of art, driving through the countryside, or maybe just stretching your arms after a long night's sleep. Who can say?

ABOUT THE AUTHOR

A PRACTITIONER NOT just of medicine but of the philosophy of health, Howard Murad, M.D., focuses on overall well-being rather than spot treatment of individual conditions or diseases. The objective of his Connected Beauty approach is to help people live healthier, happier, and more successful lives by reawakening the vigor and creativity of their youth. Following his own advice, Dr. Murad recently launched a second career as an artist. The spectacular paintings seen throughout this book are his own. Dr. Murad is the author of *The Water Secret* and *Conquering Cultural Stress* as well as the *Health and Happiness* and *Surviving Cultural Stress* series.